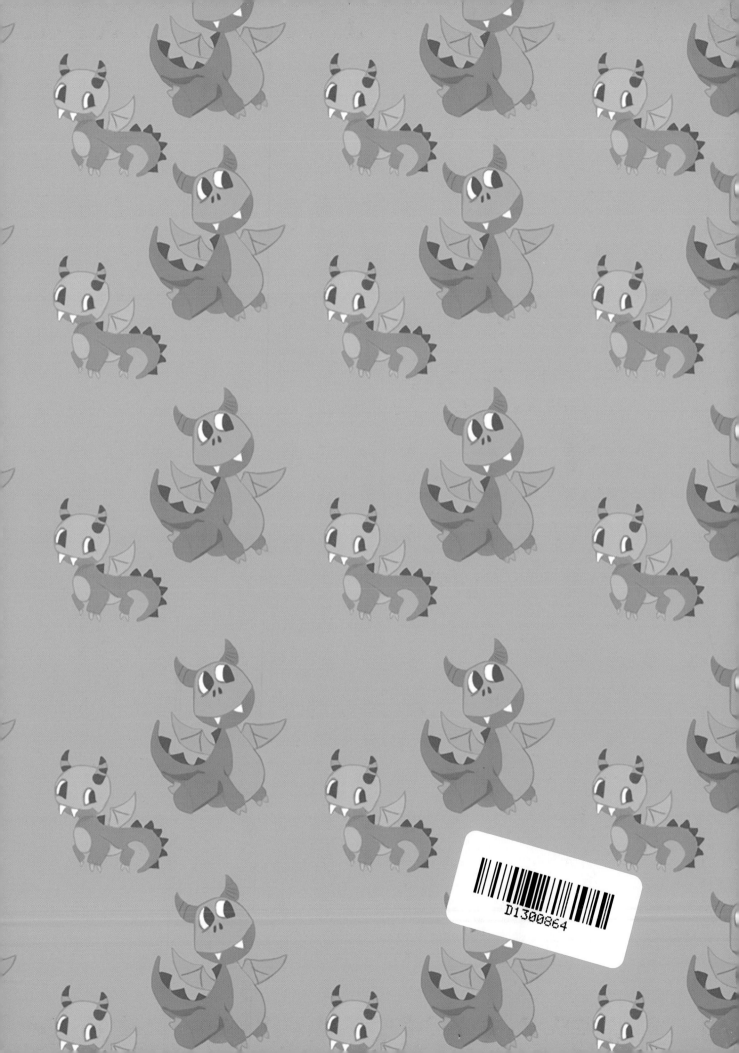

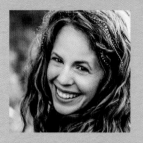

Aurora Whittet started out as a wild red-haired girl in Minnesota dreaming up stories for her friends to read. Today, she has completed *Bloodmark*, *Bloodrealms*, and *Bloodmoon* of the Bloodmark Saga trilogy and started her journey into children's books with *Mama's Knight* in honor of her own mother who lost her battle with cancer. She's a national award-winning graphic designer in her day job. Aurora lives with her family in Minnesota.

themamavillage.com | aurorawhittet.com
facebook.com/generationsofkindness | twitter.com/aurorawhittet | instagram.com/aurorawhittet

Special thank you: To my fearless editor, Amy Quale; you inspire everyone around you. Thank you for all that you do and all that you are.

ISBN 13: 978-1-94576-908-5

Library of Congress Catalog Number: 2016912517
Printed in the United States of America
First Printing: 2016

20   19   18   17   16   5   4   3   2   1

Cover and interior design by Aurora Whittet.
Illustrations by Aurora Whittet

Published by W. I. Creative Publishing, an imprint of Wise Ink Creative Publishing.

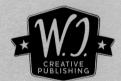

W.I. Creative Publishing
837 Glenwood Avenue
Minneapolis, Minnesota 55405
wiseinkpub.com

To order, visit **themamavillage.com**. Reseller and bulk discounts available.

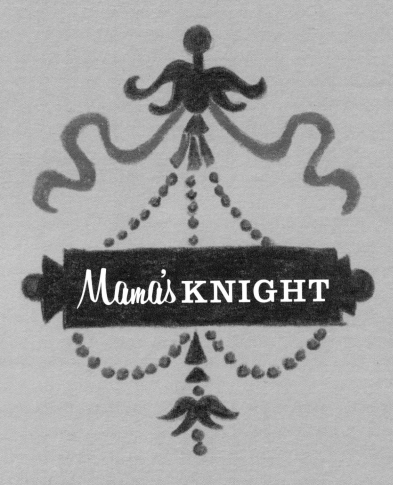

Mama's KNIGHT

AURORA WHITTET

With love for Tyson Cuever, the most valiant and true of warriors;

To my beautiful mother, who taught me how to be a mom with grace and humor. Even now that you're gone, Mom, I still feel your love all around us;

And to all the cancer *warriors*, *survivors*, *fighters*, and *caregivers* everywhere and the tiny people they love. Together, our hearts beat as one.

Once upon a time, in the great
big world, lived the most
incredible child named . . .

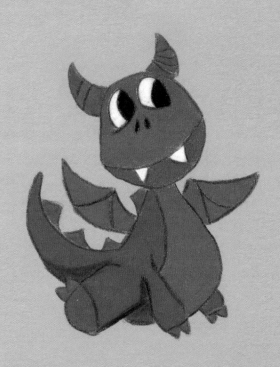

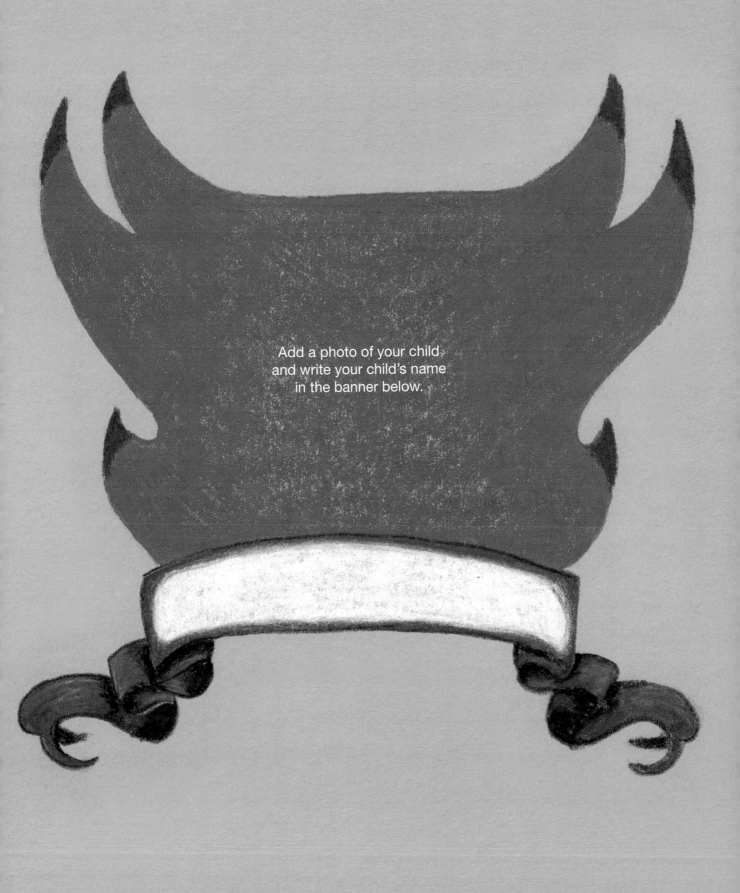

Add a photo of your child
and write your child's name
in the banner below.

Knight _____ loved
(CHILD'S NAME)
all kinds of things, like _____,
_____, and _____.

Knight _____, this is the
(CHILD'S NAME)
beginning of an epic journey with
me, your mama, across the vast
world against perilous evil. But
because of you, this journey will also
be filled with love and hope.

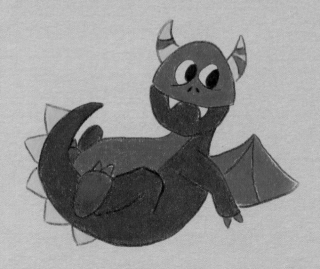

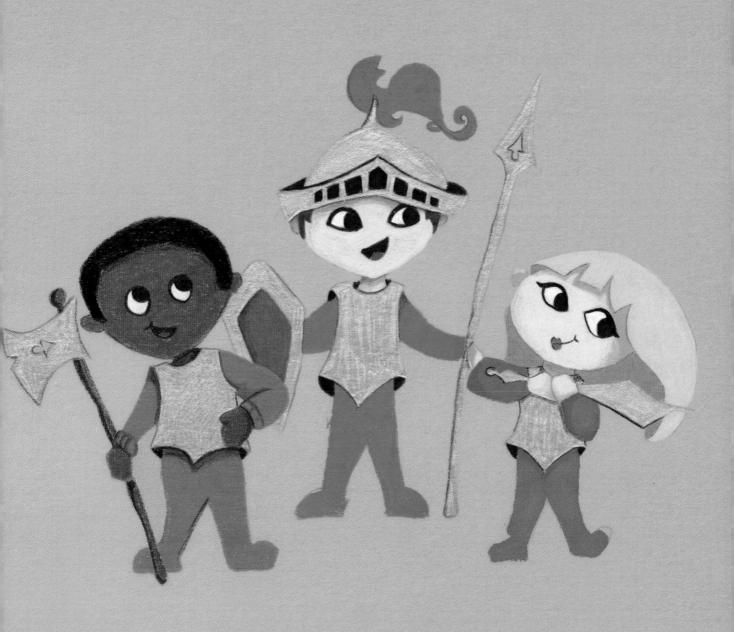

It all started one simple day when
I found out I had

cancer.

That one word felt heavier
than an elephant!

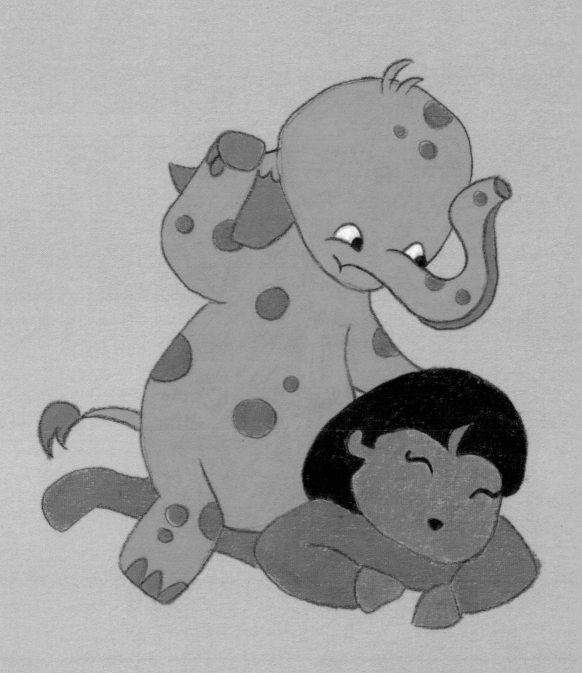

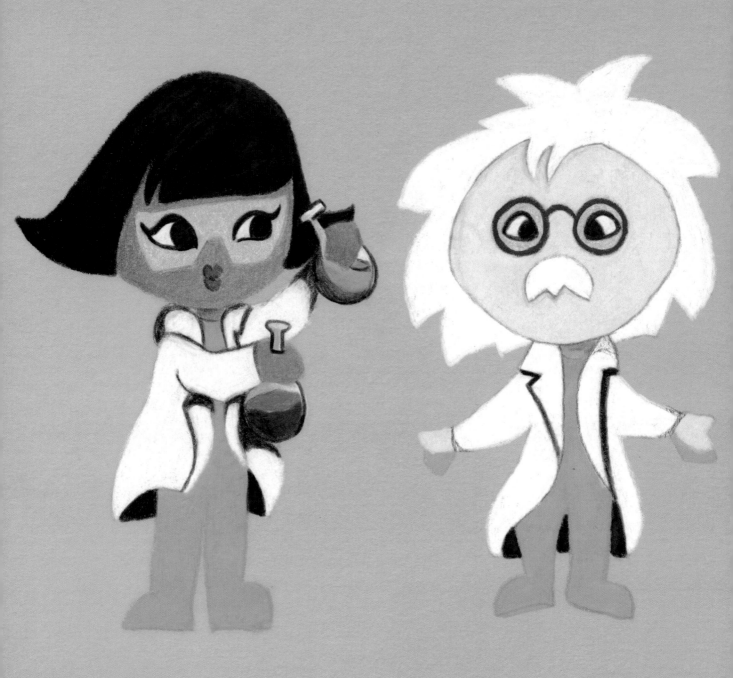

I met with some doctors,
the very best

master
geniuses

in the world, and a plan was hatched.
My treatment plan is:

_____

_____

_____

Though plans may change over time,
these are some of the medicines that
are going to help me fight:

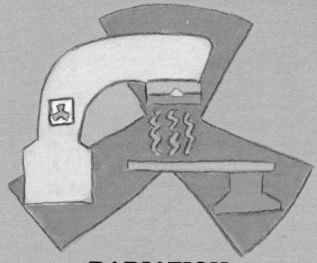

RADIATION

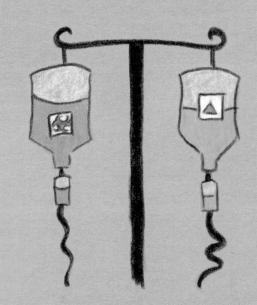

CHEMOTHERAPY

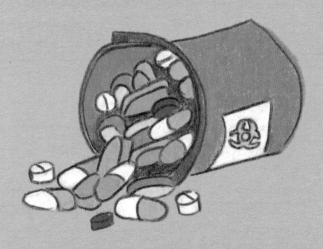

ORAL MEDICATION

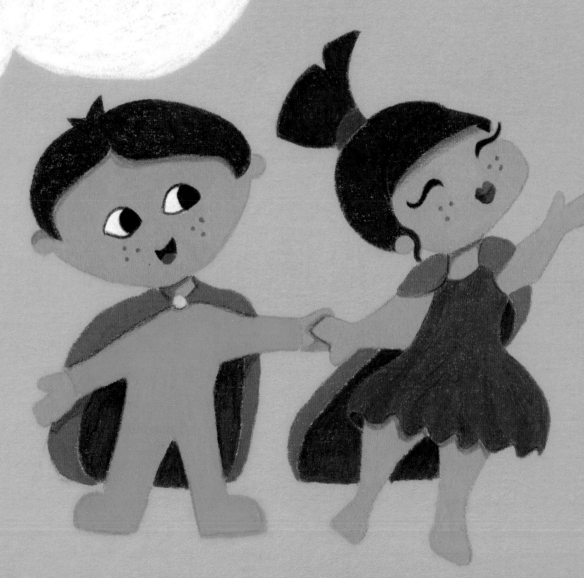

Make your own cape! Download the pattern at:
themamavillage.com/project/cape

Cancer is like a million tiny evil monsters in my body, and I have to fight them off.

It's like a valiant sword fight wages inside me!

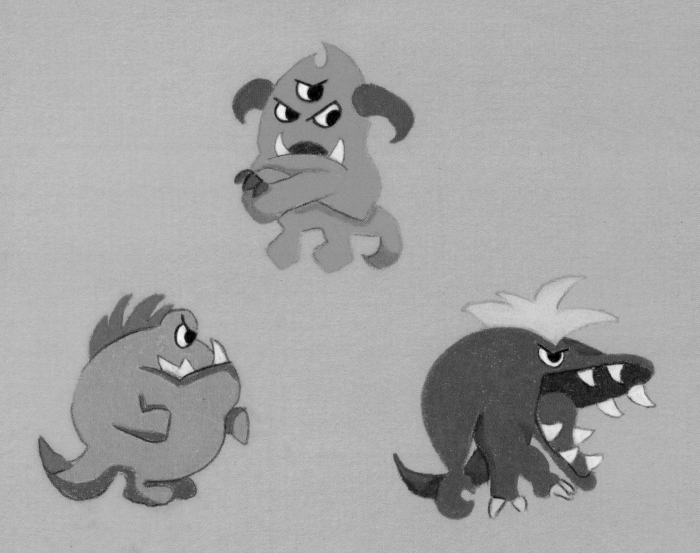

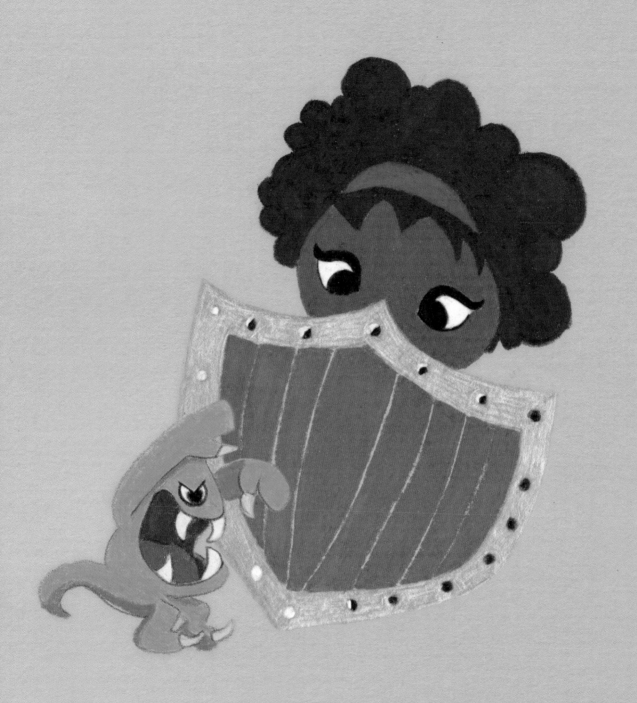

My medicines are helping me kick
cancer's butt and **you** are the knight
that I fight for every day.

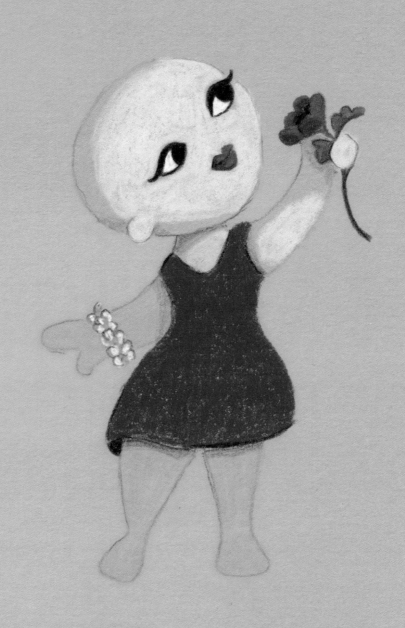

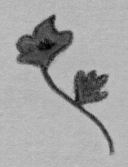

Some of my symptoms may be . . .

_____

_____

_____

_____

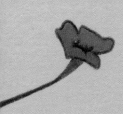

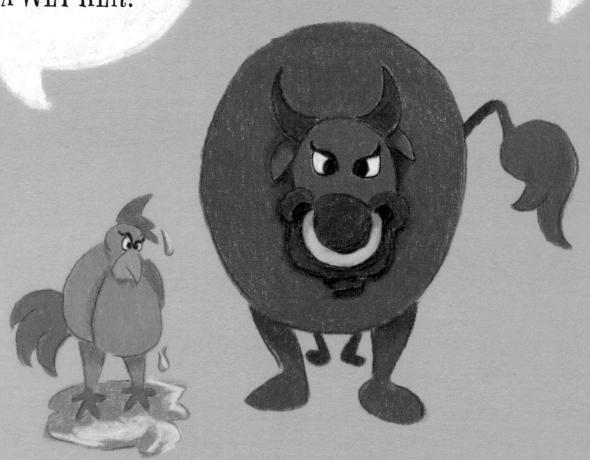

Cancer can make me tired,
frustrated, and angry.

HOW DO *You* FEEL TODAY?
LET'S TALK ABOUT IT.

MAD AS A WET HEN

NERVOUS AS A
BUTTERFLY IN A NET

AFRAID AS A
VAMPIRE AT SUNRISE

INPIRED AS A
HUMMINGBIRD

ANGRY AS A GOOSE

ENRAGED AS A BULL

LETHARGIC AS A BEAR

FURIOUS AS A FAIRY

CONFUSED AS A COW

SICK AS A CAT WITH A
HAIRBALL

ANXIOUS AS
A LITTLE DOG

NAUSEATED
AN OCTOPUS

FORGETFUL AS
MY MOM

MISCHIEVIOUS
AS A TODDLER

COOL AS A CUCUMBER

DISAPPOINTED AS
A SPORTS FAN

THANKFUL AS A DOG

GUILTY AS A FOX

CRUSHED AS
A MOUSE

POWERLESS AS A
TURTLE ON ITS BACK

SUSPICIOUS AS
AN ALLEY CAT

TERRIFIED AS A BUG

CONCERNED AS A FROG

STUPIFIED AS
A ZOMBIE

IRRITATED
AS A GOAT

FIERCE AS A
DRAGON

BRAVE AS A WOLF

OPTIMISTIC
AS AN OWL

SADDER THAN A
HUNGRY PANDA

DESPERATE AS
A HYENA

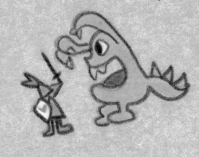

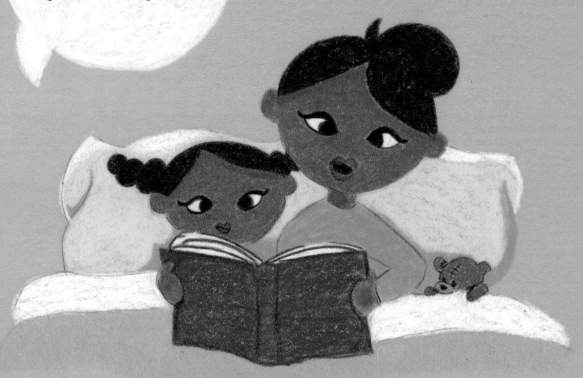

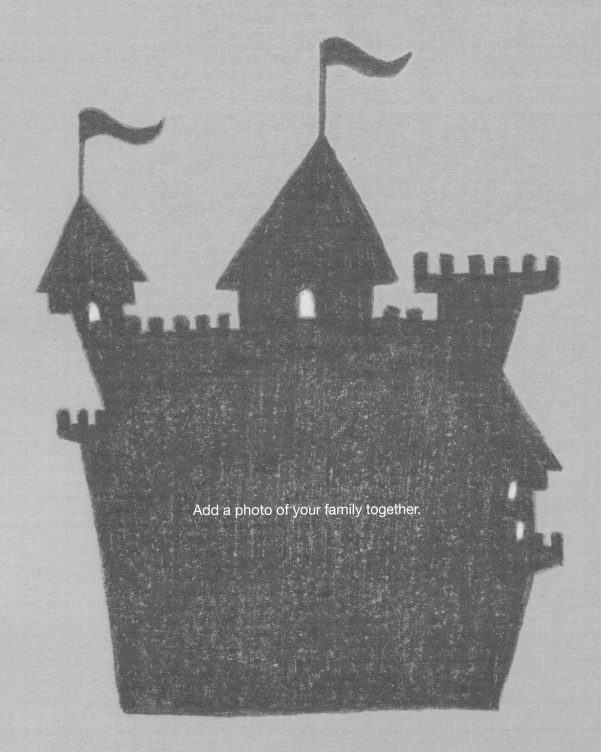

Add a photo of your family together.

But this is what makes me happy!

_____

_____

_____

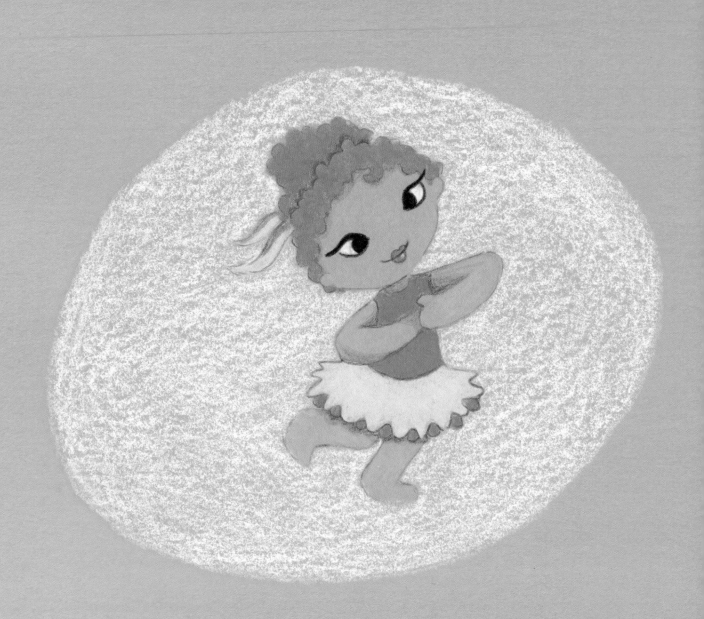

Sometimes, I need a break.
But I promise you will never
be ignored or forgotten. I even
find you in my dreams.

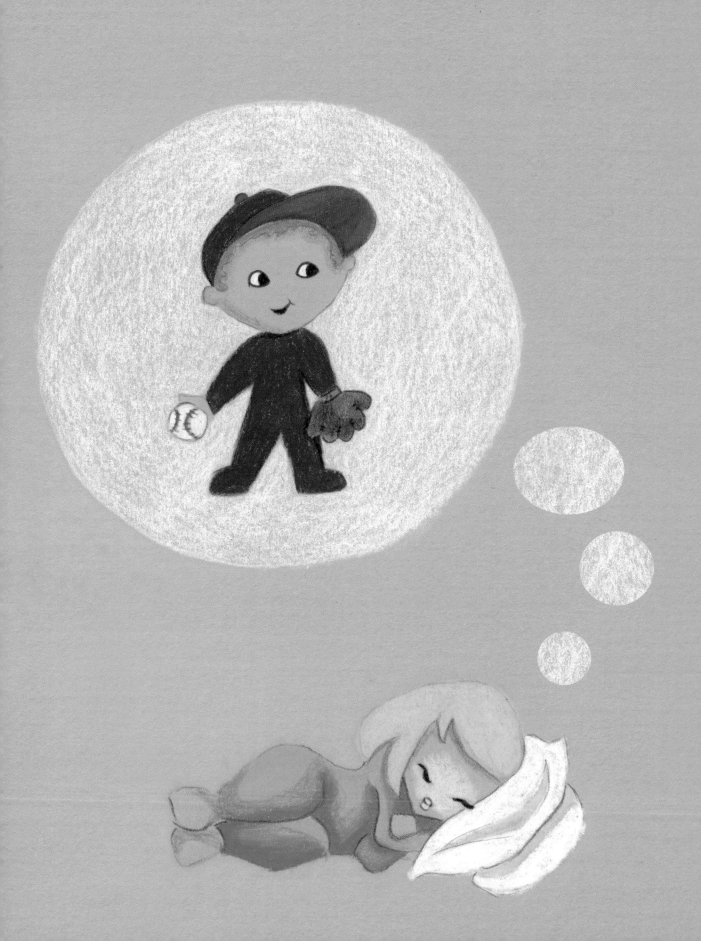

Sometimes, my body is weak
and I can't run and play or even
pick you up, but I have an idea!
Why don't we . . .

ACTIVITIES CENTER

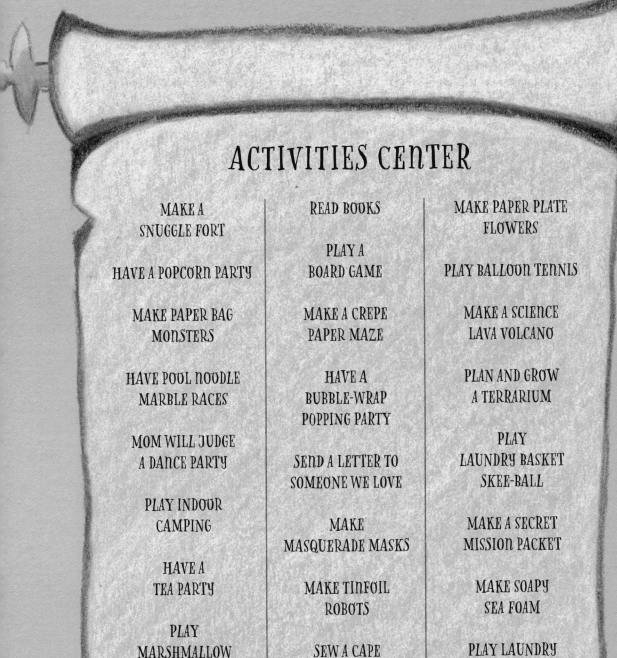

MAKE A SNUGGLE FORT	READ BOOKS	MAKE PAPER PLATE FLOWERS
HAVE A POPCORN PARTY	PLAY A BOARD GAME	PLAY BALLOON TENNIS
MAKE PAPER BAG MONSTERS	MAKE A CREPE PAPER MAZE	MAKE A SCIENCE LAVA VOLCANO
HAVE POOL NOODLE MARBLE RACES	HAVE A BUBBLE-WRAP POPPING PARTY	PLAN AND GROW A TERRARIUM
MOM WILL JUDGE A DANCE PARTY	SEND A LETTER TO SOMEONE WE LOVE	PLAY LAUNDRY BASKET SKEE-BALL
PLAY INDOOR CAMPING	MAKE MASQUERADE MASKS	MAKE A SECRET MISSION PACKET
HAVE A TEA PARTY	MAKE TINFOIL ROBOTS	MAKE SOAPY SEA FOAM
PLAY MARSHMALLOW LAUNCHERS	SEW A CAPE OR AN APRON	PLAY LAUNDRY BASKET PIRATES
MAKE DREAM CATCHERS	HAVE AN INDOOR SCAVENGER HUNT	PLAY COTTON-SWAB DARTS

Pick an activity on this chart that sounds fun!
For activity instructions, go to: **themamavillage.com/activities**

Sometimes, I feel sick
as an octopus
with the flu

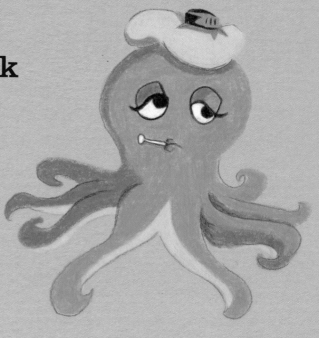

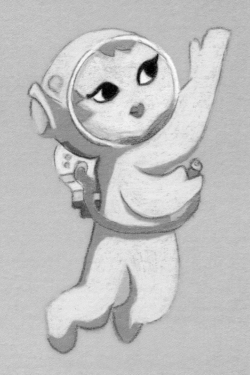

or as weak as if I
had jumped all the
way to the moon.

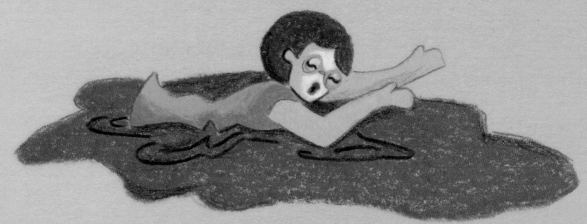

I can feel like I'm dragging myself
through a pond of sticky ooze
to get to you.

Sometimes, my favorite foods even smell like farts and I gag, but here are some things I still like:

GAG-PROOF FAMILY RECIPIES

FROM THE KITCHEN OF _____

_____

_____

_____

_____

_____

GAG-PROOF FAMILY RECIPIES

FROM THE KITCHEN OF _____

CHOOSE 3 THINGS
FROM THE CHART AND LET'S MAKE UP
A *story* TOGETHER!

_____

_____

_____

_____

_____

_____

_____

_____

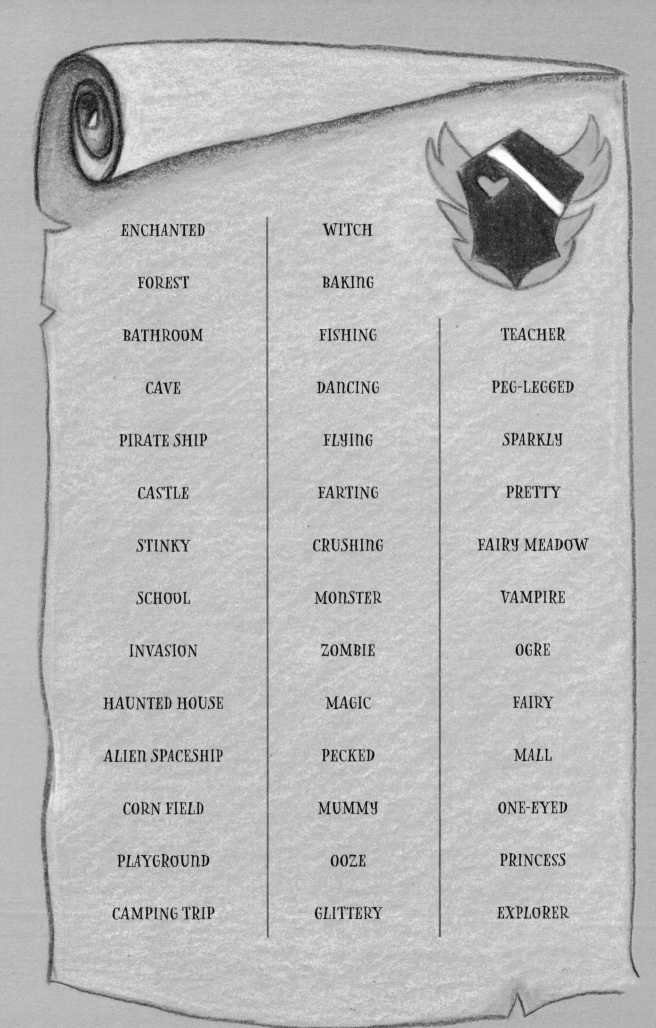

ENCHANTED	WITCH	
FOREST	BAKING	
BATHROOM	FISHING	TEACHER
CAVE	DANCING	PEG-LEGGED
PIRATE SHIP	FLYING	SPARKLY
CASTLE	FARTING	PRETTY
STINKY	CRUSHING	FAIRY MEADOW
SCHOOL	MONSTER	VAMPIRE
INVASION	ZOMBIE	OGRE
HAUNTED HOUSE	MAGIC	FAIRY
ALIEN SPACESHIP	PECKED	MALL
CORN FIELD	MUMMY	ONE-EYED
PLAYGROUND	OOZE	PRINCESS
CAMPING TRIP	GLITTERY	EXPLORER

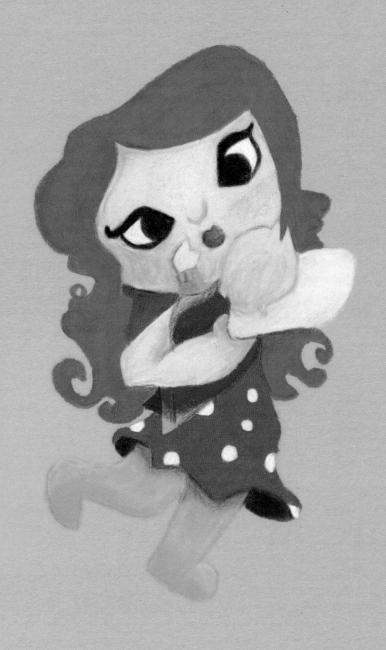

I may be sick for now, but cancer
is NOT stronger than
my love for you.

HERE IS A LITTLE SECRET
JUST FOR YOU TO KEEP.

_____

_____

_____

_____

_____

_____

If today I'm not my strongest,
or I'm feeling a bit green, let's call
for superhero reinforcements!

Fill out the coupons and let's pick
someone to come help us with
an activity of your choice.

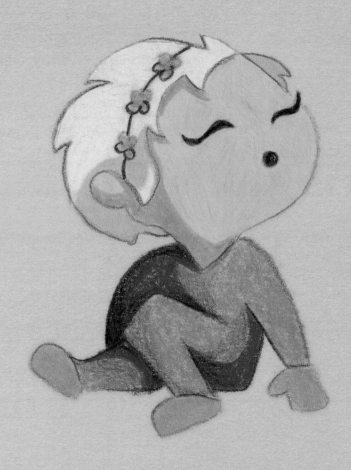

YOU ARE HERE BY DUBBED

Knight _____
(NAME OF SUPER HERO HELPER FOR THE DAY)

ON A RESCUE MISSION TO

_____
(ACTIVITY CHOSEN)

_____
(CHILD'S SIGNATURE)

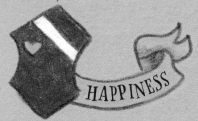

YOU ARE HERE BY DUBBED

Knight _____
(NAME OF SUPER HERO HELPER FOR THE DAY)

ON A RESCUE MISSION TO

_____
(ACTIVITY CHOSEN)

_____
(CHILD'S SIGNATURE)

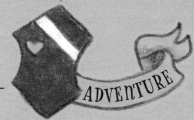

YOU ARE HERE BY DUBBED

Knight _____
(NAME OF SUPER HERO HELPER FOR THE DAY)

ON A RESCUE MISSION TO

_____
(ACTIVITY CHOSEN)

_____
(CHILD'S SIGNATURE)

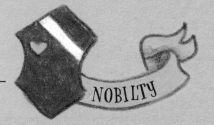

YOU ARE HERE BY DUBBED

Knight _____
(NAME OF SUPER HERO HELPER FOR THE DAY)

ON A RESCUE MISSION TO

_____
(ACTIVITY CHOSEN)

_____
(CHILD'S SIGNATURE)

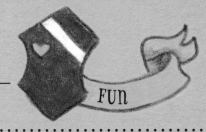

YOU ARE HERE BY DUBBED

Knight _____
(NAME OF SUPER HERO HELPER FOR THE DAY)

ON A RESCUE MISSION TO

_____
(ACTIVITY CHOSEN)

_____
(CHILD'S SIGNATURE)

YOU ARE HERE BY DUBBED

Knight _____
(NAME OF SUPER HERO HELPER FOR THE DAY)

ON A RESCUE MISSION TO

_____
(ACTIVITY CHOSEN)

_____
(CHILD'S SIGNATURE)

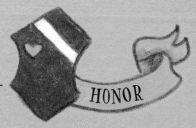

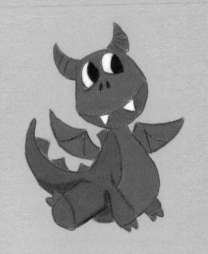
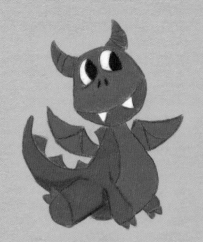
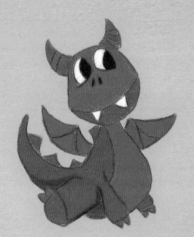
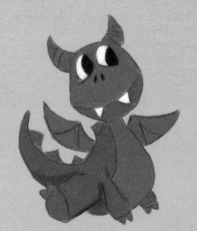
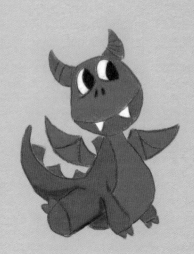
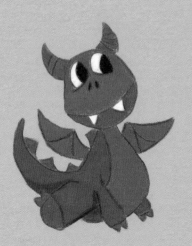

Sometimes, I'm scared,
but looking at you helps
scare all the bad away.
Like the time you . . .

_____

_____

_____

_____

_____

_____

ADVENTURES WITH MAMA

_____

_____

_____

_____

_____

_____

_____

_____

_____

_____

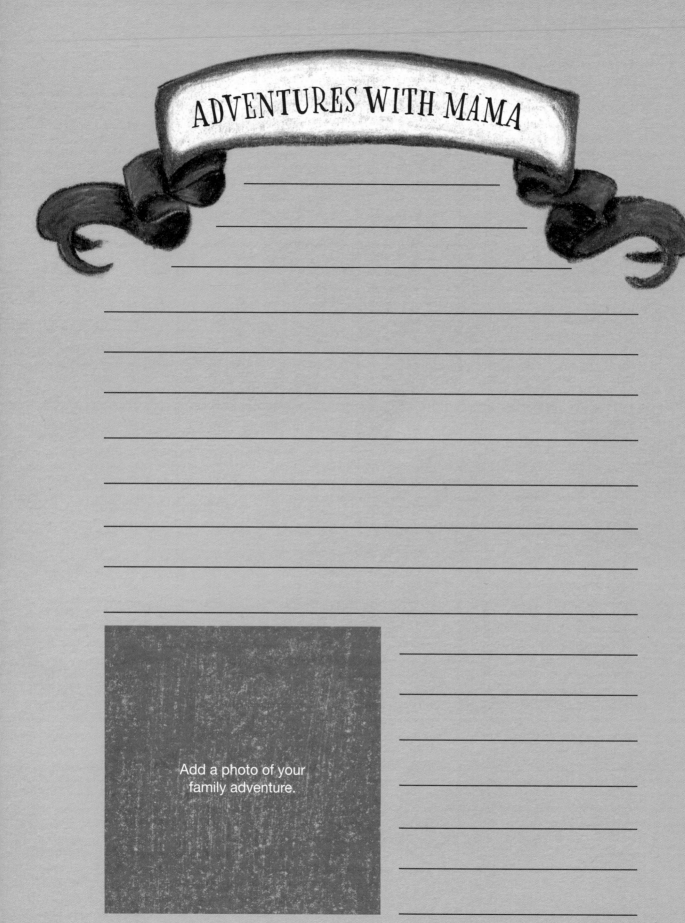
Add a photo of your
family adventure.

_____

_____

_____

_____

_____

_____

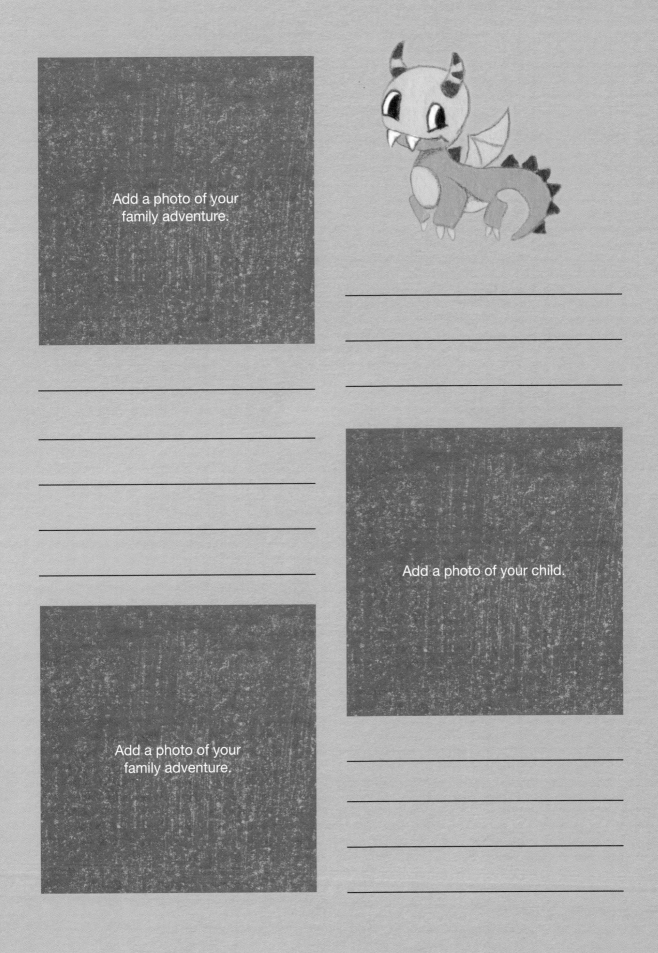

Add a photo of your family adventure.

Add a photo of your child.

Add a photo of your family adventure.

Though my cancer is scary,
I fight for you, and I am here
for you when you get scared.
I love you from your smelly toes to
your cute nose forever and always,
for you are my favorite.

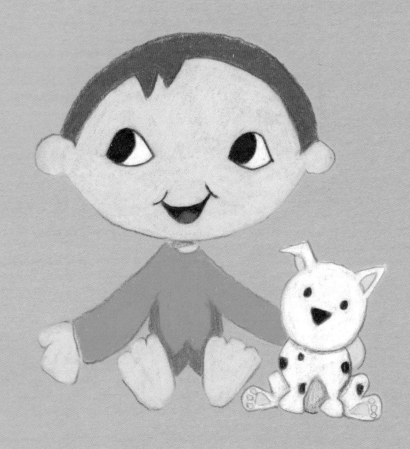

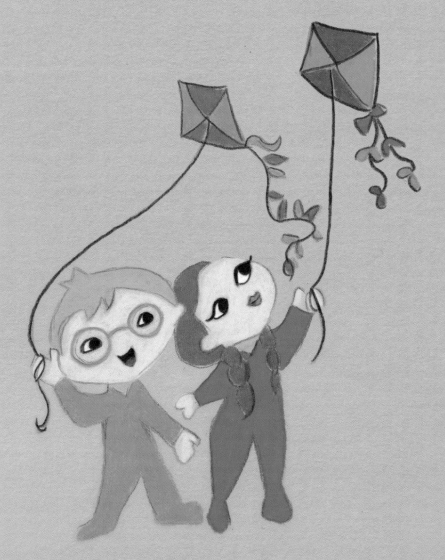

I cherish every moment that I
am given with you. And if there
is a day that we must live apart,
all you have to do is close your
eyes and feel the wind, because
I will always surround you
with my love.

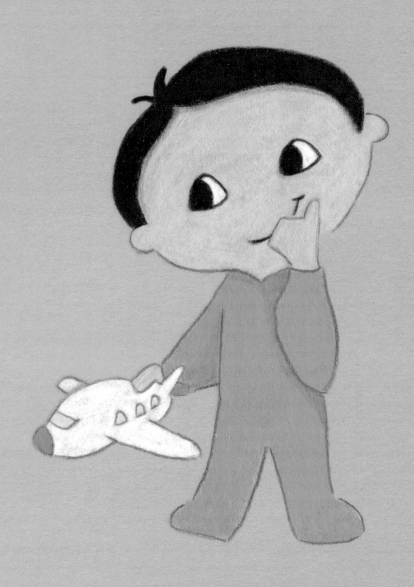

So what adventure
shall we have today?

Remember, we are never alone
on this journey—many hearts
walk with us.

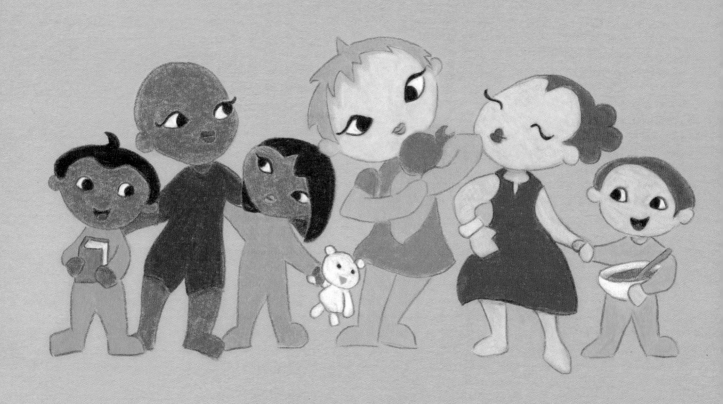

— TINY *Knights* OF HONOR —

Layla Best	Kael Cluever	Jyderian West
Abbey Brown	Leif Cluever	Lucas Wetzel
Jedidyah Brown	Will Martin	Mason Wetzel
Wyatt Brown	Isabella Peatrowsky	Henry Whittet
	Edward Ramales	

— THE *Courageous* MAMAS —

Amber Langford-Brown	Teri Dittmer	Nancy Simpson
Francie Levitt Byington	Faith Henderson	Laurie Wetzel
Tyson Cluever	Jodi Leabo	Barbara Wick
	Stephanie Mabbott	
	Sandra Showalter	

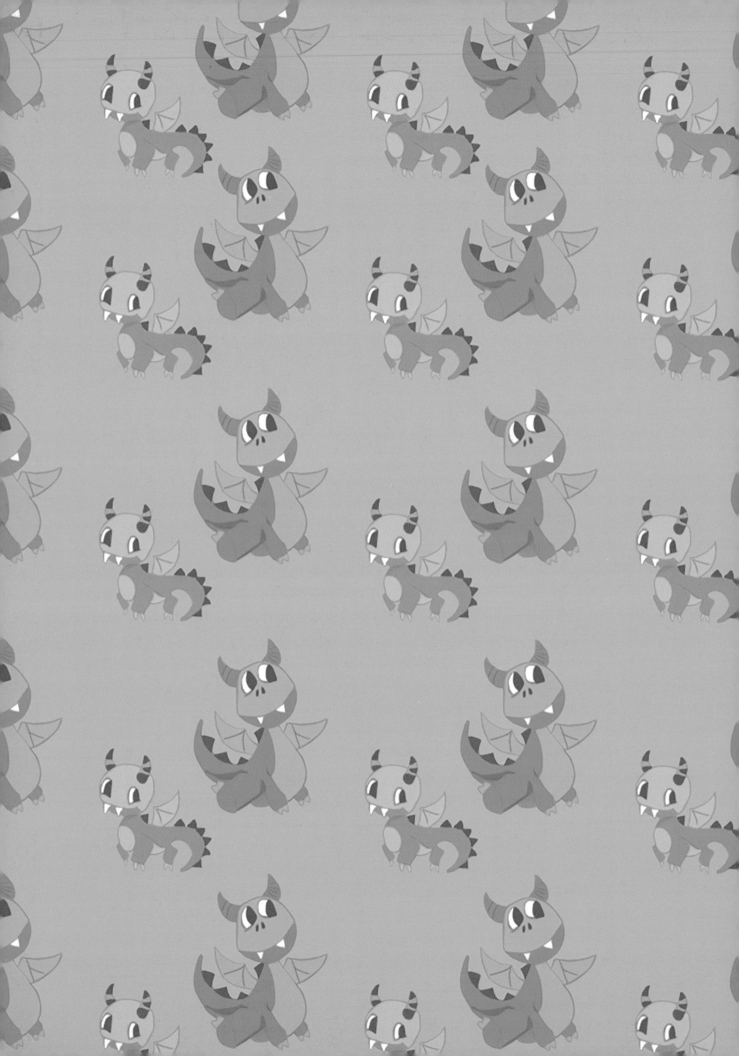